REDUCE FATTY LIVER DISEASE WITH HERBAL MEDICINES

Terry Lemerond

and

Dr. Lexi Loch

The purpose of this book is to educate. It is not intended to serve as a replacement for professional medical advice. Any use of the information in this book is at the reader's discretion. This book is sold with the understanding that neither the publisher nor the author has any liability or responsibility for any injury caused or alleged to be caused directly or indirectly by the information contained in this book. While every effort has been made to ensure its accuracy, the book's contents should not be construed as medical advice. To obtain medical advice on your individual health needs, please consult a qualified healthcare practitioner.

Reduce Fatty Liver Disease with HERBAL MEDICINES

www.TTNPublishing.com

Library of Congress Control Number: 2023909208
Print ISBN: 978-1-952507-36-6
eBook ISBN: 978-1-952507-37-3

Editor: Michele Olson
Design: Kristy Frisque
Formatting: Alt 19 Creative

Printed in the United States of America

This book is dedicated to all the true health seekers in the world.

Contents

PART 1

Your Liver-What Can Go Wrong and Why

CHAPTER 1
The Liver-Your Body's Multi-Tasker

Your liver is the multi-tasker of your body. You might even think of it as the COO—Chief Operating Officer – because it has so many functions essential to life itself that it's hard to keep track of them all.

In fact, the human liver, the largest internal organ in your body, performs more than 500 critical jobs, ranging from janitorial services like removing toxins from your bloodstream, making bile to help break down and metabolize food, to storing energy for later, and strengthening your immune system.

Even after reading just these two paragraphs, we're sure you're already wondering if there is any function of the human body that doesn't have at least some connection to the liver.

Indeed, this three-pound, football-sized organ on the upper right side of your abdomen is so crucial to your body's overall function that you will die within a week if it fails.

Liver Functions

Here's a partial list of crucial liver functions:

- Helps your body use nutrients and necessary medicines, plus excretes harmful ones
- Breaks down, balances and creates nutrients the body needs for survival and optimal health
- Activates the immune system to capture and clear bacteria, viruses, and other pathogens
- Helps produce proteins from amino acids that can be used for growth and maintenance of virtually every body tissue
- Produces bile, which:
    - Breaks down and helps the body absorb fats and fat-soluble vitamins
    - Helps excrete excess cholesterol
    - Clears bilirubin from the body, which is a by-product in the breakdown of abnormal or aged red blood cells
- Removes toxins:
    - Clears pathogens (bacteria, viruses, fungi) from the bloodstream
    - Clears heavy metals from the body
    - Clears pesticides, insecticides, industrial chemicals, and other harmful substances
    - Clears alcohol, drugs, and medications
- Metabolizes proteins, carbohydrates, and fats
- Activates enzymes for optimal digestion

- Stores glycogen (a form of glucose), vitamins, and minerals for use when needed
- Regulates hormone levels by breaking down or transforming excess hormones, including:
    - Insulin that regulates blood sugars
    - Sex hormones that control body shape and sexual function, including estrogen and testosterone
    - Thyroid hormones that control metabolism
    - Cortisone and adrenal hormones that regulate stress response
    - Aldosterone that controls fluid balance
- Balances cholesterol levels
- Helps blood clot normally
- Regulates the amount of blood in your body

This is only a bare bones synopsis of the liver's wide-ranging functions, but we're sure you get the message: The health of your liver is connected to almost every other function of your body. If you have any type of liver disease or dysfunctin, it can and will affect your entire body.

A Deeper Dive

Let's take a deeper dive into a few of these essential body functions ruled by the liver.

Sex hormones: Many of us think that sex hormones like estrogen and testosterone (there are many more, by the way) are solely a part of sexual desire and conception.

Yes, indeed, that is true, but the sex hormone estrogen is intimately (pun intended) connected not only with the overall health of the reproductive organs, but also with the urinary tract, heart and blood vessels, bones, breasts, skin, hair, mucous membranes, pelvic muscles, and brain function.

You may be surprised to learn that men produce a considerable amount of estrogen in their testes, even though women produce far more estrogen overall.

The opposite is also true: Both sexes produce testosterone, although men produce more of this particular sex hormone than women. Testosterone is essential to the formation of healthy red blood cells, strong bones and muscles, reducing insulin resistance (to prevent diabetes), and supporting energy and stamina.

In the coming chapters, you'll see how important regulating sex hormones is to the entire body. A healthy liver positively affects almost every bodily function connected to hormones. An unhealthy liver causes hormonal shortfalls that can lead to a cascade of health problems.

Detoxification:

The liver is a soldier assigned to do battle for the health of the entire body. Think of it as the body's primary filtration system. If you use drugs (whether pharmaceuticals needed to treat a specific condition or recreational), or you drink an excessive amount of alcohol, your liver is standing by to clean out the toxins.

When you are exposed to a virus (like SARS-CoV-2 [COVID], the flu or even a common cold), a harmful bacteria (like pneumococcal pneumonia, an infected cut, or food poisoning), toxic substances like air pollution, pesticides or insecticides, or even toxic food additives like glyphosate RoundUp™ in wheat products, your liver will be your first, second and third line of defense.

When the liver detects an attack of any sort, it activates specialized cells, called Kupffer cells, that work as the first line of defense to identify, digest, clean up, and sweep out any type of toxins.

In addition to the resident Kupffer cells, vitamins B and C, amino acids, magnesium, sodium bicarbonate, and glutathione are essential parts of the liver's defensive team.

Cholesterol:

We're frequently told that we should constantly worry about our cholesterol levels and yes, it's true that excessively high cholesterol, when combined with inflammation, can lead to a wide variety of health problems, like heart disease. However, your body needs cholesterol at healthy levels to thrive.

Your liver produces almost all the cholesterol you need to make strong cell membranes, many hormones, and vitamin D, an essential hormone-like nutrient that is involved in hundreds of body functions.

The organ uses one type of sugar, called fructose, to make fat. Too much refined sugar and high-fructose corn syrup causes a fatty buildup that can lead to liver disease.

In fact, if you do not obtain enough cholesterol through your diet, the liver will grab what it needs from other fats, sugar and proteins. No, this doesn't mean you should go overboard and eat a dozen eggs every day to ensure your cholesterol levels are high enough. Most of us get more than we need from the highly processed fats in our diets and alcohol consumption.

If you eat more cholesterol than your body needs, a healthy liver will take up the slack and flush out what is not needed.

Finally...

The liver is a really tough and resilient organ. Even though the liver is subjected to many unfavorable lifestyle choices, it retains the remarkable ability to repair itself, up to a certain point. Like any other organ, a lifetime of disregard for healthy lifestyle choices can—and will—eventually lead to liver dysfunction, failure and even death.

What You Need to Know:

The liver controls a vast array of bodily functions that are essential to life. More than 500 liver functions have been identified including:

- Detoxifying the body by identifying, neutralizing, and sweeping out harmful substances
- Producing or transforming protein molecules from amino acids for growth and maintenance of virtually every body tissue
- Producing appropriate amounts of cholesterol for cellular health and the production of essential nutrients while removing excess cholesterol
- Regulating estrogen, testosterone, insulin, thyroid, stress hormones, and many others that maintain balance in the body.

CHAPTER 2
Liver Diseases

As noted in the first chapter, the liver is an incredibly tough organ. It's also an incredibly versatile organ with a vast array of functions.

But, like every other organ in the human body, it's not invincible. And when things go wrong, they can go terribly wrong.

Let's start with a snapshot of the health of your liver.

In general, an annual visit to your healthcare practitioner may include certain lab tests to assess your general health.

Some tests will look at your liver's effectiveness in producing protein and clearing bilirubin, a substance that can help measure how well the liver is clearing toxins and other waste from your system.

Other tests can help monitor whether your liver is responding to disease or injury. They can screen for infections, like hepatitis B and C; they can measure the severity of liver damage, if any, and monitor the progression of these diseases.

There are eight liver tests that your doctor may (or may not) order. Not all of these tests may be ordered initially, but if abnormalities are found, it's likely your healthcare provider may explore further.

Here's the Basic List:

- **Alanine transaminase (ALT), is** an enzyme found primarily in the liver that helps convert proteins into energy for the liver cells. High ALT levels may indicate liver damage.
- **Aspartate transaminase (AST), is** an enzyme that helps metabolize amino acids. Elevated AST levels may indicate heart, liver, muscle, or kidney damage.
- **Alkaline phosphatase (ALP),** an enzyme found in the liver and bones, and is important for breaking down proteins. High levels may indicate liver damage or disease, like a blocked bile duct or certain bone diseases.
- **Albumin and total protein.** Albumin is one of several proteins made in the liver. Low levels may be a sign of liver disease or damage, and a diminished ability to fight infections.
- **Bilirubin** is a substance produced during the normal breakdown of red blood cells. High levels of bilirubin can cause jaundice

(yellowing of the eyes and skin), which can be a symptom of liver damage or disease, or certain types of anemia.

- **Gamma-glutamyltransferase (GGT), is** an enzyme found in the blood. High levels may signal liver or bile duct damage.
- **Lactate dehydrogenase (LDH),** is an enzyme found in almost all the body tissues, including the liver. High levels may indicate liver damage, but it can also signal many other disorders like kidney disease, pancreatitis, heart disease, and some types of cancer.
- **Prothrombin time (PT), measures** the time it takes your blood to clot. Prolonged PT may indicate liver damage because the liver is not making the correct amount of blood clotting proteins. However, PT can also be prolonged if you're taking certain blood-thinning drugs, such as warfarin.

Acute Liver Failure (ALF)

Sudden liver failure is life threatening. In fact, 20% of people with the condition do not survive. Those who do survive can have significant consequences such as brain damage and multiple organ failure.

So how does your liver fail suddenly?

Acetaminophen (most common brand name: Tylenol) overdose is the most common cause of acute liver failure in the Western world.

While intravenous N-acetyl-cysteine (NAC) may be lifesaving if given within eight hours of the overdose, ALF may not be diagnosed that fast. Then a liver transplant may be the only treatment.

Acetaminophen overdose is the leading cause for calls to Poison Control Centers. It is the cause of more than 56,000 emergency room visits, 2,600 hospitalizations and 500 deaths due to acute liver failure each year in the U.S. It accounts for about half of all acute liver failure cases in the U.S., which can also be caused by poison, some medications and cancer, among other causes.

While the maximum daily dose for control of pain and inflammation is 4,000 mg per day for adults, ALF has occurred in people taking considerably less than that, usually following the advice of their doctors.

This isn't news. We've known for more than 20 years that even recommended doses of acetaminophen can be fatal, yet they remain on the market, supporting a deadly billion-dollar industry. Please avoid taking acetaminophen whenever possible. There are safe and effective natural alternatives for pain and fever.

Chronic Liver Disease

Liver Infections

You've probably heard of hepatitis, a type of liver infection that is most often caused by a virus. There are at least six different types of viral hepatitis. This section will focus on the three most common types of viral hepatitis (A, B, and C) that can cause inflammation and potentially serious liver disease.

Hepatitis A:

You know those signs in restaurant restrooms that say all employees should wash their hands with soap and water after using the toilet? That's because hepatitis A is caused by a foodborne virus that can spread to food or drinks through the feces of an infected person. You may even feel compelled to wash your hands right now.

Hepatitis A isn't very common. The Centers for Disease Control and Prevention (CDC) says there are around 25,000 cases in the U.S. every year. There are vaccines available and most people who get hepatitis A usually recover in a few weeks or months, without serious liver damage. Death from the disease is rare and happens most often in people who are weakened by other serious diseases.

Hepatitis B:

Primarily spread through the bodily fluids (blood, semen) of infected people, hepatitis B is a serious disease that can lead to liver cancer. You can contract hepatitis B from sexual contact with an infected person, sharing needles or other medical equipment (including glucose monitors) with an infected person, even sharing toothbrushes or razors. Babies born to an infected mother are at high risk of developing hepatitis B.

The biggest problem with hepatitis B is that there are hundreds of thousands of people who are infected and don't know it. The CDC estimates that 862,000 Americans are living with hepatitis B. The worldwide incidence of the disease is staggering: There have been about two billion cases of hepatitis B since testing began in 1971 and 300 million are chronically infected today, according to the Hepatitis B Foundation. About 1.5 million new cases are diagnosed every year, but only about 10% of the people with the disease know they have it, so it can spread like wildfire. Hepatitis B vaccines are readily available. Untreated hepatitis B can have dire and even deadly consequences, as we'll investigate in the coming pages.

Hepatitis C:

Spread through contaminated blood, hepatitis C is the most common form of viral hepatitis, causing about 50,300 acute cases in the U.S. each year. An estimated 2.4 million of us are living with a hepatitis C infection.

About half of the people who have the disease are unaware they have it since there are few, if any, symptoms in most cases and it can sometimes take decades for symptoms to appear. You can get hepatitis C through blood transfusions, shared needles or medical equipment. Contaminated blood can be received through transfusions, organ transplants before 1991 (when testing became mandatory) and poor infection control in medical facilities. It can also be passed from mother to baby.

Hepatitis C is the primary cause of liver disease that can lead to the need for liver transplants. It can also cause liver cancer.

There is no vaccine for the disease, but there are treatments that can clear chronic hepatitis C infections from the body in 90% of cases.

Non-Alcoholic Fatty Liver Disease *(NAFLD)*

Experts at Mayo Clinic call Non-Alcoholic Fatty Liver Disease (NAFLD) "an umbrella term that applies to a range of liver conditions that affect people who drink little or no alcohol." Translation: NAFLD is caused by a buildup of fat in and around the liver so the liver can't function properly.

More translation: In general, almost all cases of NAFLD are caused by insulin resistance, type 2 diabetes, and obesity. and particularly to the accumulation of belly fat. If you or someone you love is carrying extra weight, particularly in the abdomen, be aware that this could lead to serious liver disease.

What happens when you eat refined sugar and high fructose corn syrup? The liver uses excess fructose to create fat, a process called lipogenesis.

Excess consumption of sugar and simple carbohydrates is a major contributor to obesity, so healthy eating choices are a first big step toward protecting yourself against obesity and NAFLD.

You'd probably be shocked to learn that NAFLD is the most common liver disease in the U.S., about one-quarter—yes, that's 25%!—of all Americans having some form of this disease.

NAFLD is a complex disease that merits its own chapter. Please read on to the next chapters for a deeper dive into NAFLD and natural ways you can prevent or reverse it.

Cirrhosis

Cirrhosis is a late-stage liver disease in which healthy liver tissue becomes stiff and scarred. It's a "progressive" disease, meaning that all of the other liver issues mentioned in this chapter can deteriorate into cirrhosis. With cirrhosis, healthy liver tissue is replaced with scar tissue, inevitably impairing a multitude of liver functions. There are many stages of cirrhosis. It is typically considered irreversible, although some newer evidence is contradicting this long-held theory. Nevertheless, if you've been diagnosed with cirrhosis, you can make lifestyle changes that may slow the progress of the disease and lengthen your life expectancy.

About 4.5 million American adults have cirrhosis. It kills about 70,000 of us a year, a number that is gradually increasing because of the obesity epidemic and its intimate connections with NAFLD that can progress to cirrhosis.

Here are the main causes of cirrhosis of the liver:

- Obesity and metabolic disorders
- Alcohol abuse
- Type 2 diabetes
- Drug use with shared needles
- History of liver disease, including hepatitis
- Unprotected sex
- Some chronic diseases like hemochromatosis, Wilson's disease, and cystic fibrosis

The diabetes-cirrhosis connection is a question of the chicken or the egg: About 30% of people with cirrhosis have type 2 diabetes and 96% have some glucose intolerance, according to Mexican research. But researchers concluded that it's unclear whether cirrhosis is caused by diabetes alone or by metabolic syndrome, a basket of symptoms including insulin resistance, high blood pressure, high cholesterol and triglycerides, and excess body fat, all of which almost inevitably accompany type 2 diabetes.

What's abundantly clear is that long-term heavy drinking and alcohol abuse are high-risk behaviors that frequently result in cirrhosis, long-term illness and death. It is estimated that cirrhosis is present in up to 25% of people with any alcohol-related disorders, including abuse, dependence, addiction, and alcoholism.

What's equally clear is that excess fat surrounding organs, whether it's visible or not, is not only a major cause of NAFLD, but of cirrhosis and a wide variety of other diseases. For anyone with metabolic disorders, like insulin resistance, obesity and type 2 diabetes, please discuss nutrition and lifestyle strategies with your healthcare practitioner.

Stages of Cirrhosis

There are two basic stages of cirrhosis: compensated and decompensated.

Many people with hepatitis and other liver diseases don't show any symptoms until liver damage is extensive.

Compensated cirrhosis is asymptomatic, meaning that there are no obvious signs of the disease. Because it's asymptomatic, you may not suspect cirrhosis is present unless you undergo regular testing.

We'll be straightforward with you here: If you drink more than two alcoholic drinks a day, if you have had any form of hepatitis, or if you have excess weight around your waist, *please* get an annual liver panel.

Signs and symptoms of cirrhosis indicate decompensated (deadly) cirrhosis may include:

- Yellow discoloration in the skin and eyes (jaundice)
- Swollen legs, feet or ankles (edema)
- Extreme fatigue
- Easy bleeding or bruising
- Nausea
- Loss of appetite
- Unexplained weight loss
- Dark colored urine
- Itchy skin

Treating Cirrohsis

There is no cure for cirrhosis. The majority of the damage done to your liver is permanent. However, depending on the underlying cause of your cirrhosis, there may be actions you can take to keep your cirrhosis from getting worse, including:

- Immediately stop drinking alcohol
- Treat chronic hepatitis (if you have it)
- Eat a healthy, well-balanced, minimally processed diet that includes avoiding sugar and simple carbs

- Avoid medications that stress the liver, including statin drugs, acetaminophen, antivirals, anabolic steroids, and many others. Medications should be discussed with your healthcare practitioner before adding or discontinuing them
- Start a botanical regimen that may slow progression

Cirrhosis also increases the risk of liver cancer.

People with cirrhosis may qualify for a liver transplant, but those organs are scarce. Only 9,236 liver transplants were conducted in the U.S. in 2021. You can run the numbers. That means that only about 13% of people who have end stage cirrhosis will get transplants. The rest will die.

We know that sounds grim. It *is* grim.

Prevent Liver Disease

Prevention is the best route. We said it a couple of pages back and we'll repeat it because this is so important: If you've ever had any type of liver disease, treat it and have your liver function checked annually. Make the lifestyle changes that can prevent deterioration into cirrhosis. Your life quite literally depends on it.

Your best prevention strategy if you have never been diagnosed with any type of liver disease:

- **Drink alcohol in moderation.**
  For healthy adults, that means up to one drink a day for women and up to two drinks a day for men. Heavy or high-risk drinking is defined as more than eight drinks a week for women and more than 15 drinks a week for men.

- **Risk reduction.**
  Use a condom during sex. If you choose to have tattoos or body piercings, be vigilant about cleanliness and safety when selecting a shop. Seek help if you use illicit intravenous drugs, and don't share needles to inject drugs.

- **Discuss vaccination with your healthcare provider.**
  If you're at increased risk of contracting hepatitis or if you've already been infected with any form of the hepatitis virus, talk to your doctor about getting the hepatitis A and hepatitis B vaccines.

- **Use medications wisely.**
  Take prescription and nonprescription drugs only when needed and only in recommended doses. Don't mix medications and alcohol. Talk

to your doctor before mixing supplements with prescription or nonprescription drugs.

- **Avoid contact with other people's blood and body fluids.**
  Hepatitis viruses can be spread by accidental needle sticks or improper cleanup of blood or body fluids.

- **Keep your food safe.**
  Wash your hands thoroughly before eating or preparing foods. If traveling in a developing country, use bottled water to drink, wash your hands and brush your teeth.

- **Limit chemical exposure.**
  If you need to use chemical-based products, do so in a well-ventilated area, and wear a mask when spraying insecticides, fungicides, paint, and other toxic chemicals. Always follow the manufacturer's instructions.

- **Protect your skin.**
  If you must use insecticides and other toxic chemicals, wear gloves, long sleeves, and a hat and mask so that chemicals aren't absorbed through your skin.

And above all—

- **Maintain a healthy weight. Abdominal fat is a key risk factor for NAFLD and other metabolic diseases. Weight loss can help reduce your risk and even reverse NAFLD.** Aim for daily exercise, blood sugar and cholesterol balance, and a nutrient-dense, whole-foods diet that avoids sugar and simple carbs.

What You Need to Know:

Liver disease can be caused by:

- Excessive alcohol consumption
- Obesity
- Viral infections like hepatitis A, B or C
- A few chronic diseases like hemochromatosis, cystic fibrosis, and autoimmune diseases

Liver diseases, if left untreated, can deteriorate into cirrhosis, that will cause liver failure, require a liver transplant if one is available (only 13% of terminally ill cirrhosis patients get a transplant each year), and death if poor lifestyle choices continue.

To prevent and slow the progression of liver diseases:

- Drink alcoholic beverages moderately or not at all
- Lose weight if you are overweight
- Treat hepatitis if you have it. If you don't know, get tested
- Get regular blood tests to track liver function
- Practice safe sexual behavior, including barrier methods and testing
- Do not share needles or any medical or personal hygiene devices.

CHAPTER 3
Non-Alcoholic Fatty Liver Disease

There's good news and bad news here.

First the bad news: Non-Alcoholic Fatty Liver Disease (NAFLD) is reaching epidemic proportions, along with type 2 diabetes, obesity and metabolic syndrome, conditions that are all linked.

The good news: In its earlier stages, NAFLD is reversible when nutrition, exercise, and stress management are prioritized. For instance, a 10% weight reduction—that's just 20 pounds if you weigh 200 pounds!—will stop the liver disease in 90% of all NAFLD cases, provided that the weight loss is long-term.

More bad news: If it's not addressed, NAFLD can deteriorate and eventually become cirrhosis of the liver. You know from Chapter 2 that this is a serious, irreversible disease that will affect every part of your life.

There are two basic types of NAFLD—simple fatty liver sometimes called NAFL and Non-Alcoholic Steatohepatitis (NASH). At the risk of overwhelming you with medical terminology, NASH is the more serious problem because in about 15% of cases, it causes liver inflammation and eventual scarring (fibrosis) that leads to cirrhosis, the serious and incurable condition that leads to liver failure.

Research shows that obesity is a major risk factor for type 2 diabetes. A major link between these two conditions is insulin resistance, along with chronically elevated blood sugar levels and diets high in processed fats. These risk factors also help tie the thread between obesity and NAFLD. All of these risk factors are serious for children as well, where we are seeing similar trends in the rising levels of both NAFLD and obesity. More on kids and NAFLD in the coming pages.

Obesity Epidemic

Let's take a detour for a moment and investigate the obesity epidemic in the United States.

The numbers are frightening. In the U.S., 41.9% of the adult population is classified as obese, according to the Centers for Disease Control and Prevention (CDC). Let that settle in for a minute: Of our population of approximately 332 million, 139 million of us are obese. Add in those who are overweight, but not yet classified as obese, and the number rises to a staggering 236 million, 71% of the entire population! Obesity has multiple causes, among them poor nutrition, harmful lifestyle choices, environmental toxins and genetic predispositions, but the numbers are still quite shocking.

These significant increases in body mass have occurred primarily over the past three decades. What has changed so much in that time period? Easier access to high-calorie, high sugar, highly processed foods, combined with sedentary lifestyles and increasing amounts of environmental toxins (typically stored in fat cells) can slow your metabolism. These drastic increases in obesity are connected to the way our food is grown, produced, processed and saturated with chemicals; the high cost of organic foods vs. the low cost of processed foods. Limited access to healthcare, financial inequality and nutritional and educational shortfalls, are also factors.

Researchers generally define obesity by body mass index (BMI), a somewhat flawed measure calculating a ratio of height and weight. What's wrong with BMI? It doesn't take into account lean muscle mass, which is heavier than fat. It also doesn't consider gender, age or ethnicity. Nevertheless, it is a measure generally accepted in the medical profession and can at least be considered a snapshot of general health.

This means if you are an "average" 5'4" American woman who weighs 170 pounds, you're considered overweight. You've just slid under the classification of obese. At 145 pounds, you'd be considered at the upper edge of a healthy weight. An "average" 5'9" man would squeak into the healthy category at 168 pounds, but the average weight for his height would be 198 pounds.

Obesity rates are higher for women in general, especially as women age. They are even higher for low-income, non-white women who live in the Midwest or the South, according to the CDC.

And body size is getting bigger and bigger, almost by the year. The CDC says that between 2000 and 2020, the American obesity rate increased from 30.5% to 41.9%. Worse yet, the number of severely obese Americans, once called morbidly obese, nearly doubled from 4.7% to 9.2%. Obesity rates also increased during the pandemic, likely caused by sedentary behavior, high stress levels (job insecurity or loss, uncertainty from the pandemic, etc.), isolation and other factors that make it difficult to maintain a healthy diet and lifestyle.

Add in children: The obesity epidemic has snowballed in the past 20 years. The CDC reports that 19.7% of American children under 19 are obese. Add in overweight kids and the figure rises to 35%. That means our kids have major health risks, including type 2 diabetes, something that was virtually unknown in children until about 25 years ago.

We're sure you get the point. We won't sugar coat it (pun intended): Most of us carry excess weight, including fat around our organs that prevents them from functioning optimally, creating a high risk for NAFLD.

What is it costing us? It's costing us our lives. Medical science has known for decades that excess weight causes type 2 diabetes, heart disease and strokes, joint problems and—you guessed it, the subject of this book— liver dysfunction.

They're all tied together in a complex ball. Who knows which one starts the cascade toward serious health problems, but we can tell you that very few people are connecting excess weight with the prospect of serious liver problems and the devastating healthy consequences that can accompany them. If we did, it might help us choose water instead of sugar-sweetened beverages, reduce our consumption of simple carbohydrates, and move our bodies daily.

The Consequences

With the obesity epidemic numbers engraved in our brains, it's time to look at the ways metabolic disorders, like obesity, are affecting our livers.

NAFLD was briefly mentioned in Chapter 2 when we talked about liver diseases. This perilous disease is the most common liver disease in the Western world. Worse yet, most of the people who have NAFLD have no symptoms and they have no idea how serious that excess abdominal fat (and hidden fat around the organs) can be.

The American Liver Foundation estimates that about 25% of the American population has NAFLD. Wow! That means 85 million of us have this buildup of fat in our livers that is easily preventable, easily reversible (up to a point) and potentially fatal if we do nothing about it. For us, that's another big WOW!

The National Institute of Diabetes and Digestive and Kidney Diseases (NIDDK) cites research that estimates that 75% of overweight people and 90% of obese people have NAFLD.

NAFLD is the most common cause of chronic liver disease in children in the United States. Studies suggest that 5% to 10% of all children have NAFLD. The disease has become more common in children in recent decades, largely because childhood obesity has become so prevalent.

The Mayo Clinic warns that NAFLD usually causes no signs and symptoms in children or adults, which explains why it is probably underdiagnosed. When it does cause symptoms, they may include fatigue and/or pain, or discomfort in the upper right abdomen.

The NIDDK says 20% to 50% of children with NAFLD have the more serious form of the disease, called NASH. That is directly related to the obesity epidemic among children and our propensity for sugary drinks and fast-food meals.

Possible signs and symptoms of NASH and advanced scarring (cirrhosis) include:

- Yellowing of the skin and eyes (jaundice)
- Chronic fatigue
- Abdominal swelling (ascites)
- Enlarged blood vessels just beneath the skin's surface
- Enlarged spleen
- Red palms
- Chronic fatigue
- Extreme skin itching (pruritus)
- Abnormal brain function (encephalopathy)

Diabetes

Type 2 diabetes was once called Adult-Onset Diabetes, because it rarely occurred in people under 50. Now it has become common in children and teenagers. Why? I'm sure you guessed it: highly processed foods and beverages that can lead to metabolic disorders, like the obesity epidemic.

Obesity is a common factor in type 2 diabetes and NAFLD. About 10% of the adult American population has been diagnosed with type 2 diabetes. The number is much lower among children, about 4.1 per thousand but it's growing dramatically as our lifestyle choices deteriorate. That number has nearly doubled since 2000.

Worse yet, experts agree that these numbers are probably much higher since many people do not know they have the disease.

Diabetes is bad enough on its own. We've known for decades that people with type 2 diabetes are at higher risk for heart disease and strokes, blindness, amputations, and cancer. Now we have to add liver disease to that sad list.

With kids and adults alike, it's estimated that type 2 diabetes reduces a person's life expectancy by about six years. The decrease in quality of life is anybody's guess.

It's all worse, much worse, when it comes to kids. Just imagine a ten-year old child diagnosed with type 2 diabetes. By the age of 40, they will already be suffering the side effects of diabetes that once were reserved for octogenarians (people in their 80s) if they live that long.

About 70% of people of all ages with type 2 diabetes also have NAFLD.

As we mentioned before, the relationship between NAFLD, NASH and type 2 diabetes is a chicken and egg question. Which came first? We don't know for sure, but we do know that people with type 2 diabetes are at an extremely high risk of developing NAFLD, NASH, and cirrhosis. People with NASH are highly likely to have type 2 diabetes as well. What we do know for sure is that controlling type 2 diabetes with diet, exercise, and antidiabetes medications or supplements also helps decrease the severity of liver diseases.

Lean NAFLD

Yes, it's possible for thin people to have NAFLD (and type 2 diabetes). In fact, a 2018 study shows that about 7% of Americans with NAFLD are considered "lean" or "non-obese."

Researchers aren't exactly sure why this is the case, but they theorize that some thin people can have similar profiles for metabolic diseases, like diabetes and heart disease, as overweight and obese people.

It's also possible for people with a normal BMI to have abdominal fat (and/or fat around their organs) even though they may appear thin.

The Inflammation Factor

Inflammation is a factor in almost all disease processes, ranging from heart disease to diabetes to cancer. And yes, metabolic diseases, like obesity and NALFD are inflammatory conditions.

If you are obese, or have diabetes, heart disease, Alzheimer's, osteoporosis, depression or cancer, you have a disease triggered by unresolved, chronic inflammation. If you don't have any of these diseases yet, count yourself lucky, be proactive about it and do what you can to prevent or minimize your levels of inflammation.

One of the reasons obesity is dangerous is because excess fat cells release proteins, in the broad category called cytokines, that produce low level inflammation, which can persist for a long time, even decades. If the inflammation continues unchecked, it disrupts many biological functions, including the immune system, metabolism, and yes, liver function. Most people have no symptoms of long-term inflammation. It often goes completely unnoticed until an inflammatory disease begins.

Treatment

This is the really bad news: There is no conventional medical treatment or pharmaceutical intervention to reverse liver disease. In some cases, the liver damage stops or even reverses itself, with weight loss or other lifestyle changes. But in other cases, NAFLD, NASH and cirrhosis will be a permanent fixture in the patient's life.

You can stop and possibly even reverse NAFLD by:

- Reducing weight, especially around the abdomen
- Controlling blood pressure and cholesterol
- Controlling type 2 diabetes
- Avoiding alcohol
- Avoiding over-the-counter pain relievers, especially acetaminophen
- Avoiding refined sugar and high fructose corn syrup products.

Stay with us. There are a number of things you can do and some time-tested botanical remedies that can help protect your liver, and, if you have any form of liver disease, they can help stabilize and even minimize the seriousness of the disease.

What You Need to Know:

- The dramatically increasing rates of obesity and excess weight in the United States are a major risk factor for the increasing rates of liver disease in adults and children.
- NAFLD and NASH often go hand-in-hand with type 2 diabetes. Obesity is often a common link between the two.
- Losing weight can stabilize or even reverse NAFLD. NASH and cirrhosis are irreversible, but they can be stabilized with the right lifestyle choices.

CHAPTER 4
How You Can Achieve a Healthy Liver

The best way to fight liver disease is not to get it at all! But if you do have challenges to your liver, it may not be too late.

We've said in the previous chapters that most liver diseases are the result of lifestyle choices. The good news is that healthy lifestyle choices can reverse NAFLD and, if more serious liver disease like NASH or cirrhosis have come into your life, you can stabilize your liver function and prevent deterioration.

At the risk of sounding like cheerleaders, we're on your side. You are in charge.

We suspect you've tried numerous ways to bring about a healthier lifestyle. You've probably had successes and failures. What is a failure anyway, except a chance to learn?

Our point here is that you know yourself best. In this chapter, we're going to give you some options. Some you may already know and some you may not have considered. We're confident that one or two or ten of them will resonate with you and these will be your keys to success.

Since our primary focus here is on NAFLD, we can't tap dance around the issue of obesity. So, what is a healthy diet? There is so much information and misinformation out there (especially on the Internet), it's not surprising if you are confused.

There is no one diet that will promote liver health just as there is no single one eating plan that will guarantee weight loss.

However, there is one thing for certain: Sugar is the culprit in almost all disease processes, including obesity and NAFLD. Refined sugar and high fructose corn syrup cause fatty buildup that leads to liver disease. Research confirms that sugar can be as damaging to the liver as excess alcohol consumption.

We hate to harp on this so much, but it is crucial: Eliminate sugar and simple carbs (white flour products, rice, pasta and pastries for starters) from your life and you will be much healthier.

Here's a personal discovery: Eating even a little bit of refined sugar triggers cravings that are hard to rein in. Instead, get your sweetness from fresh fruit, small amounts of honey and even healthier no-calorie sweeteners like stevia.

Liver Health Eating Plans

Here are the basics:

- Banish refined sugar and high fructose corn syrup from your eating plan.
- Limit your carbohydrate intake to a maximum of 50 g daily.
- Eliminate processed foods that often have hidden sugar, sodium and unhealthy fats.
- Eat moderately. Most of us eat far too much.
- Include healthy oils like olive, macadamia nut, avocado, and pecan.
- Include healthy fats in organic butter and cream.
- Consider going gluten free.
- Avoid rapid weight loss. Shedding a pound a week is ideal. Losing more than 3.5 pounds a week can cause further liver stress.
- Stay hydrated with plenty of water and herbal teas, especially green tea.

Nutrition Plans To Consider

Let us start by saying that we're not fans of the idea of "dieting." We'd prefer to explore "eating plans" that are structured to promote a lifetime of healthy eating.

If you've struggled with your weight, you know exactly what we mean. You may try a particular diet, initially lose some weight, but over time it can become more difficult to adhere to the (often restrictive) diet, and the weight that was lost may return, and then some. That's because the concept of "dieting" implies deprivation and a temporary change. We're looking for lifelong, permanent change for our own health and longevity, and specifically for liver health.

Liver Health Eating Plans

Here's a basic rule of thumb:

- Banish refined sugar and high fructose corn syrup from your eating plan.
- Aim to reduce simple carbohydrate intake, which can quickly spike blood sugars. For those following a ketogenic diet this may be 50 grams or less per day of carbs.
- Eliminate processed foods that often have hidden sugar, sodium, and unhealthy fats.
- Focus on eating meals that leave you satisfied, without feelings of heaviness or fatigue.
- Include healthy oils like olive, macadamia nut, avocado, and pecan.
- Include healthy fats in organic butter and cream

- Consider going gluten free for a period of time and see if you notice changes in your digestion
- Avoid rapid weight loss. Shedding a pound a week is ideal. Losing more than 3.5 pounds a week can cause further liver stress.
- Stay hydrated with plenty of water and herbal teas, especially green tea.

Before we get into a synopsis of various eating plans that we think can be very successful, let us caution you to be patient. Dramatic weight loss programs are not healthy. Not only are they destined to fail, they can actually harm your liver even more than obesity. Aim to shed no more than 3.5 pounds a week, and preferably much less. A program that lets you shed about a pound a week is probably the healthiest and the kindest to your liver.

We'll also say that food plans are immensely complex. We're just giving you the bare bones summary here. We've included resources for each, so you can take a deeper dive into plans you think would work for you.

Mediterranean:

This is an eating plan based on traditional cuisines of Greece, Italy and other Mediterranean countries. It celebrates whole grains, legumes, healthy fats (think olive oil!), seafood, fruits, nuts, seeds, herbs and spices.

Animal proteins (like meat and dairy products) are included in small amounts.

This eating plan tends to avoid fried foods, sugar, unrefined grains and flour products, and excessive red meat.

A study published in the New England Journal of Medicine has shown the Mediterranean diet reduces the risk of heart attack, stroke and death related to heart problems by 30%.

Quite appropriately, Italian researchers concluded that the Mediterranean diet is the most effective for people with NAFLD: "[The] Mediterranean diet has been recommended as the best dietary pattern since it is easy to follow and, independently of caloric intake, its nutritional components have beneficial metabolic effects that not only improve steatosis (NASH) but also risk factors for cardiovascular events, the leading cause of morbidity/mortality in individuals with NAFLD."

We'd add to the Mediterranean diet these specific foods that help improve liver health:

- Beets
- Radishes (Spanish black radish)
- Burdock root
- Artichokes
- Lemons
- Parsnips
- Dandelion greens
- Watercress
- Berries

Resource: https://www.healthline.com/nutrition/mediterranean-diet-meal-plan

Ketogenic:

Popularly known simply as "keto," this is an eating plan that emphasizes low carbohydrate and high fat consumption. It advocates putting your body into ketosis, a state where you burn fat for energy instead of glucose. It limits carb consumption to around 20 to 50 grams per day, includes clean and lean protein and urges you to fill up on fats, such as meat, fish, eggs, nuts and healthy oils. The plan advocates getting 75% of your daily calories from fats, which ideally should come from avocados, seeds, nuts, olive oil and other healthy, unsaturated fats.

Those who follow this eating plan conduct simple at-home urine testing to assure they are in ketosis and burning fat.

Ketosis is different from ketoacidosis, a potentially dangerous condition that can affect people with type 2 diabetes. If you have type 2 diabetes and NAFLD, which can be common in people with weight control problems, please work closely with your healthcare professional.

Resource: Ketogenic-diet-resource.com

Paleo:

This eating plan is based on what our hunter-gatherer ancestors would have eaten before humans became farmers. A modern Paleo diet includes fruits, vegetables, lean meats, fish, eggs, nuts and seeds. It doesn't include foods that became more common when small-scale farming began about 10,000 years ago, including grains, legumes, and dairy products.

The keto and paleo diets generally include more fat than protein or carbs. It's important to note here that excess carbohydrate consumption can certainly be harmful to the liver. Low fat diets can also be harmful. Some experts attribute the beginning of the obesity epidemic to the notion that low-fat diets are essential to weight loss.

"Since the 1960s, when experts started advising people to eat less fat—based on the belief that a high-fat diet led to a high-fat body—obesity has skyrocketed. Recent evidence suggests that all those years of focusing on ways to get fat out of foods has actually contributed to the obesity epidemic," according to David Ludwig, professor of nutrition at Harvard's T.H. Chan School of Public Health.

This is partly because healthy fats were replaced by sugars and highly processed foods, both of which we now know trigger weight gain.

Resource: https://thepaleodiet.com/

Intermittent Fasting:

An eating plan that switches between fasting and eating on a regular schedule, intermittent fasting focuses more on *when* you eat rather than so much on *what* you eat (within reason!) based on a concept similar to the keto diet that your body switches from burning its blood sugar stores and starts burning fat for energy, in this case when you don't eat for several hours or even for a day.

For example, you might eat only during a specified eight-hour period every day, say between 11 a.m. and 7 p.m. or you might eat only one meal two days a week.

A 2021 review of several studies on intermittent fasting and NAFLD showed that people who engaged in this eating plan lost weight, had lower BMIs and lower ALT and AST levels (you remember these blood markers for liver disease?).

Resource: https://www.healthline.com/nutrition/intermittent-fasting-guide

Our Recommendations

Here's what we think is a sensible eating plan that will be effective for weight loss *and* liver health:

- Reject refined sugar in all forms.
- Reject processed foods.

- Embrace plentiful fresh fruits and non-starchy vegetables.
- Add healthy fats, nuts and seeds.
- Enjoy whole grains without gluten.
- Focus on complex carbohydrates, rather than simple and refined carbs.
- Limit red meat, dairy and animal fats.
- Give your body an occasional rest by not eating for 16 to 24 hours once a week or so.
- Drink water, lots of it, to help your liver flush out toxins.
- Drink green tea to speed up your metabolism and decrease fat in the liver.
- Drink coffee to help reduce insulin resistance and improve the function of liver enzymes.

None of this means you will never enjoy a piece of birthday cake or indulge occasionally in a spaghetti dinner, but these should be rare treats. Enjoy them and return to your healthy plan.

Noom And Similar Plans:

We consider Noom an educational plan that can help you change your emotional relationship with food as well as give you tools for healthy weight reduction. We know many people who have been very successful with the plan that encourages self-awareness and practical advice.

We particularly like the concept of caloric density. For example, you might eat a very large salad full of greens and fresh veggies and maybe even a few ounces of protein like tuna or chicken for lunch. You will feel full and satisfied on about 400 calories.

For the same 400 calories, you could eat a small bare beef hamburger patty. You'd still be hungry and thinking about the bun and those fries and that sugary drink to fill you up.

Noom is supportive of other eating plans mentioned here. It's full of daily tips that can help you develop long-term results with weight management.

www.noom.com

Ditch the Gluten:

Here's some bad news: There is no such thing as targeted exercise to reduce belly fat. Thousands of crunches won't do the trick!

Good news: There are solutions.

Here's what we know: Gluten intolerance causes inflammation. For some people, gluten intolerance contributes to chronic inflammation that can lead to unbalanced hormones, poor digestive function, altered intestinal permeability ("leaky gut"), which are all part of metabolic disorders, like obesity. In many cases, gluten intolerance can be responsible for the abdominal fat that we struggle so hard to shed.

Celiac disease is an autoimmune response to eating gluten. While it is relatively rare, a growing percentage of Americans are prone to gluten intolerance or sensitivity, which can have symptoms similar to celiac disease.

Gluten intolerance may also be a by-product of the routine use of glyphosate (RoundUp), a known hormone disruptor used in harvesting wheat in the U.S. but banned in Europe.

Exercise

We feel that humans are designed to move, and no healthy lifestyle is complete without daily movement or exercise.

Here's the simple plan:

- Gradually build up to 150 minutes of moderate-intensity movement like brisk walking, water aerobics, light cycling, or something similar. Find one that you like and stick with it. Even better, exercise with a buddy to help keep both of you on track.
- Add in strength training for 30 to 45 minutes two or three times a week to help build muscle strength, endurance. This will increase your energy levels and improve your quality of life. Plus, it can reduce insulin resistance. Best of all, Israeli research shows

it helps people with NAFLD to reduce NASH and more serious liver disease.

- If you're not quite ready for a more energetic movement plan, try low impact exercises like yoga, Qi Gong, and Tai Chi. These practices help with balance, strength, stress reduction, and inner peace.

Don't know where to start? A couple of sessions with a personal trainer can help provide exercises that you can do at the gym or at home.

Support Your Lymphatic System

Think of the lymphatic system as the body's transport system. This network of tissues, vessels and organs works to move lymph, a colorless, watery fluid, into your bloodstream. It delivers nutrients to your cells, helps remove waste products, helps maintain fluid balance in your body, produces immune cells, absorbs fats, and transports them where they are needed.

Every day, your liver produces up to half of the 12 liters or so of lymphatic fluid in your body.

The lymphatic system is underrecognized and underappreciated. In fact, it's the only body system that does not have its own "specialist" in conventional medicine.

Enlarged and potentially malfunctioning lymph nodes are signs of infection and can also be a telltale sign of acute and chronic liver disease. Pay attention if you find a hard knob, especially in your armpit or groin that doesn't disappear in a few days.

How To Support And Improve Your Lymphatic Circulation:

- Dry skin brushing
- Castor oil packs
- Exercise
- Lymphatic massage (self-massage or with a massage therapist)
- Drink more water
- Jumping on a mini trampoline
- Breathing exercises
- Alternating hot and cold water in the shower
- Far infrared sauna
- Herbal teas

Finally...

In addition to the herbal support, we'll explore in the next section of this book, consider adding some basic supplements to help support your liver, especially while you're working on nutrition and lifestyle changes.

Nutrients To Consider:

- **Vitamin D** to help reduce overall inflammation and specifically liver inflammation
- **Omega-3 fatty acids** like those found in cold-water fish that can help reduce the accumulation of fat in the liver
- **Lecithin/phosphatidylcholine** to help improve liver function, especially in people with NAFLD
- **Glutathione** to help the liver flush out toxins
- **B vitamins** to reduce liver inflammation and scarring in people with NASH

What You Need to Know:

There is seemingly an endless stream of eating plans to help lose weight and reduce inflammation and scarring in your liver.

What's really important:

- Realize it's not a diet. You are adopting an eating plan that you can sustain for life.
- Know yourself. Choose an eating plan that you can sustain and enjoy.
- Eliminate refined sugar and high fructose corn syrup.
- Exercise is a key element of weight management. Aim for 150 minutes of movement a week and 30-45 minutes of strength training twice a week or more.
- Pay attention to the health of your lymphatic system.
- Consider liver-supporting supplements. More to come on botanicals for liver health in the next several chapters.

PART 2
Botanicals to Promote Liver Health

Non-Alcoholic Fatty Liver Disease (NAFLD) is largely impacted by nutrition and lifestyle choices. Fortunately, there are lifestyle choices that can change the course of the disease and prevent its progression to NASH and cirrhosis.

In this section, we're going to take a deeper look at botanicals that have been scientifically researched and validated as effective in treating and reversing NAFLD. It's wonderful how Mother Nature provides medicine to treat our illnesses and modern science proves their effectiveness!

CHAPTER 5
Andrographis

Andrographis *(Andrographis paniculata)*, affectionately known as the King of Bitters, is an adaptogen, one of the multi-taskers of the plant world. In the simplest possible terms, adaptogens, like andrographis, are plant medicines that help our bodies adapt to change and support longevity.

Many people use adaptogens to prevent or postpone the chronic diseases of aging, recognizing their uncanny ability to fix what's wrong, boost what's right, keep the body in balance and prevent body functions from deteriorating.

Adaptogenic powers like those we see in andrographis have been scientifically validated as effective against chronic inflammation, atherosclerosis (hardening of the arteries), neurodegenerative cognitive impairment (Alzheimer's disease and other forms of dementia), metabolic disorders, diabetes, cancer and a host of other age-related diseases, including NAFLD, NASH and cirrhosis of the liver.

Adaptogens, like Andrographis, work through many pathways to activate the body's defense system and metabolic rate that will reverse the negative physical effects of stress and restore the body back to balance and health.

Andrographis is an incredibly valuable botanical for liver protection in Ayurvedic and Traditional Chinese Medicine (TCM). It is central to the herbal traditions of several Asian countries.

In TCM, andrographis is classified as a "cold" medicine, helping rid the body of fevers, toxins, and heat. This is especially important when we look at the detoxification function of the liver.

In the Ayurvedic tradition, andrographis is similarly considered dry, penetrating and cooling.

As is often the case, the effectiveness of a medicine that has been used and revered by Indigenous Peoples for millennia is now affirmed by modern science. By the end of 2022, the National Library of Medicine's database returned 1,242 published studies on the wide spectrum of health effects of andrographis dating as far back as 1951.

Many of the substantial healing powers of andrographis come from andrographolides, a rare group of diterpenoid lactones that have strong and scientifically proven anti-inflammatory, antioxidant, and antimicrobial effects. Andrographis is also a rich source of other nutrients, including well-researched antioxidant flavonoids and polyphenols.

In fact, andrographolide is so well regarded that pharmaceutical companies are even experimenting with synthetic versions of it, a plan that will almost certainly go awry.

With this in mind, my advice is to make sure that the andrographis you add to your regimen delivers natural andrographolide. Look for a source that is standardized to at least 20% andrographolides for a concentrated level of this incredibly versatile compound.

NAFLD

A multi-national team of researchers from the U.S., South America, and Europe concluded that andrographis helps treat and reverse NAFLD by controlling the fibrosis and inflammation found in NAFLD, NASH and cirrhosis.

Andrographis has been shown to reduce fatty acid content in the liver by 33%. Research demonstrates it can reduce pro-inflammatory conditions, decrease liver enzyme values and liver fibrosis percentage, all to the benefit of your liver.

An important 2021 Chinese animal study found that andrographolides reversed AST and ALT markers in obese laboratory mice, partly because of its anti-inflammatory and antioxidant actions, plus its ability to reverse insulin resistance found in type 2 diabetes. These are two important lab tests in determining the deterioration of liver function in NAFLD and in difficult-to-reverse NASH.

Indian researchers sang the praises of andrographolides in treating NAFLD in a 2017 study that concluded, "Our results showed that (andrographolides) could be a promising lead to treat NAFLD with comparatively low toxicity and improved efficacy."

It's interesting that the Chinese and Indian studies are among only a few conducted directly on andrographis and liver protection. Hopefully that means more research will soon be underway as andrographis continues to show positive results for NAFLD and other liver conditions.

Metabolic Syndrome

Andrographis has also been extensively studied as a treatment for type 2 diabetes and cardiovascular disease. Since we know these conditions are so closely linked to NAFLD and NASH, we think it's reasonable to consider that these studies confirm the liver protective effects of andrographis.

Remember we examined metabolic syndrome in the first section of this book? This basket of high blood sugars, high blood pressure, high blood fats and excess abdominal fat is not only a recipe for type 2 diabetes and heart disease, but also for NAFLD, NASH, and cirrhosis.

Andrographis offers an answer to all the components of metabolic syndrome, especially obesity. Taiwanese and Indian researchers found that andrographis prevents diabetes and heart disease in lab animals even when they were fed a diet high in processed fats. Other researchers confirm it helps control blood sugars.

One study shows that andrographis reduces blood sugars in diabetic rats by as much as 52.9%.

Malaysian researchers found that andrographis was a valuable tool in the treatment of type 1 diabetes (an autoimmune disease where the body's immune system attacks the insulin producing cells in the pancreas, usually diagnosed in childhood or the early teens) and type 2 diabetes (once called adult-onset diabetes, characterized by the body's inability to use or respond to the insulin the body produces). This study concluded that andrographis "was found to be quite effective in restoring the disturbed metabolic profile of obese diabetic rats back towards normal conditions."

Taiwanese researchers found that andrographis helps lower fatty accumulations in artery-clogging foam cells, reducing the risk of atherosclerosis, commonly known as hardening of the arteries.

Another team of researchers from Brazil and Bangladesh found that andrographis is effective in treating and preventing cardiovascular disease and diabetes stemming from metabolic syndrome, calling andrographis a "new hope" in the treatment of metabolic syndrome.

Additionally, a 2015 clinical trial found that andrographis extract was just as effective as gemfibrozil, a pharmaceutical that reduces the amounts of fat produced by the liver in patients with elevated triglycerides (blood fats) and cholesterol. Researchers suggested andrographis might be used as an alternative medicine for high triglycerides. Gemfibrozil can have serious side effects, including muscle weakness, blurred vision, irregular heartbeat, and fatigue. Research has found that andrographis has no serious side effects.

All of this is an impressive array of scientific proof that andrographis is a powerful tool against the core diseases that can lead to NAFLD, NASH, cirrhosis and liver failure.

Antiviral

Andrographis is also well studied as an effective treatment for other liver diseases caused by a variety of viruses, including hepatitis A, B, C, D and E. It's also revered as a treatment for colds and flu and now for the SARS-CoV-2 (COVID-19) virus.

In one study, andrographis has even been shown to eliminate 80% of cases of infectious hepatitis.

In another study published in 2014, Taiwanese research shows that andrographis is an effective treatment for hepatitis C.

Researchers theorize that the potent antiviral effects of andrographis can be responsible for the successful treatment of these terrible diseases and preventing their progression to cirrhosis, liver cancer, and death.

In December of 2022, a team of Indian and Malaysian scientists concluded that andrographolides are a strong contender to treat COVID-19 infections.

There's More . . .

There is a reason why andrographis is such an important part of Asian medical traditions and why it is increasingly being researched in the Western world.

A major finding in 2011 showed that andrographis offers protection against liver damage caused by acetaminophen. You'll recall from Chapter 1 that acetaminophen poisoning can cause sudden acute liver failure and is the primary cause of poisoning deaths in the U.S.

Here's a small snapshot of the scientifically validated benefits of the King of Bitters.

It's A Constantly Changing List As Science Finds More And More Ways This Miracle Herb Works:

- colds, flu, upper respiratory infections
- virus fighting, including the herpes simplex virus
- infection fighting, including staph, salmonella and MRSA
- joint pain, arthritis
- cancer: almost all types
- malaria and other illnesses caused by parasites
- ulcerative colitis and other digestive problems
- multiple sclerosis
- Alzheimer's disease and dementia

- heart disease by lowering cholesterol and blood pressure, dissolving blood clots
- diabetes, types 1 and 2
- rheumatoid arthritis and other autoimmune diseases

What You Need to Know:

Andrographis has been used for centuries to prevent and treat a wide variety of diseases, including liver disease, in Asian medical traditions.

Research shows that andrographis and its key compounds, andrographolides:

- Reduces fatty acid content in the liver by 33%, preventing further liver damage
- Reduces inflammation and fibrosis that contribute to liver damage
- Addresses components of metabolic syndrome:
- Helps control obesity
- Reduces insulin resistance and improves blood sugar control
- Helps control high levels of blood fats (triglycerides)
- Protects against viral infections that cause all forms of hepatitis
- Addresses a broad range of other diseases including cancer, arthritis, Alzheimer's disease and more.

CHAPTER 6
French Grape Seed Extract

Meet another of Mother Nature's multi-taskers!

French grape seed extract comes from the royalty of grapes. Think of French wine and you'll quickly get the idea: There is nothing better!

Our ancestors loved making wine by fermenting grapes. Today's science has confirmed the health benefits of wine and grapes, many of which are derived from the seeds themselves. Concentrating those life-giving and even life-extending benefits of grape seeds into an extract gives us French grape seed extract (FGSE) a potent tool that should be part of every household's medicine cabinet, whether you are suffering from one of the many diseases of aging or if, like all of us, you want to avoid them altogether.

A major part of the power of *Vitis vinifera,* FGSE's botanical name, comes from substances with the tongue-twisting name, oligomeric proanthocyanidins (OPCs).

Although OPCs are found in many plants, they are concentrated to extraordinary levels in grape seeds, hence their healing power.

OPCs are probably the most potent antioxidants known to science.

Lifestyle choices and exposure to environmental toxins over a lifetime cause free radical oxygen molecules to accumulate in your cells. That free radical oxygen exposure triggers chronic inflammation, opening the door to cell aging and genetic deterioration, as well as to the diseases of aging, including cancer, heart disease, diabetes, Alzheimer's, metabolic syndrome and more. Now we are counting NAFLD in that basket of chronic diseases of aging.

At least 90% of all our modern-day diseases are caused by oxidative stress and inflammation.

Now there is something you can do to reduce oxidative stress and its disease-causing consequences: Take advantage of the healing power of FGSE.

FGSE and NAFLD

You already know that the obesity epidemic has sparked the rising numbers of Americans afflicted with NAFLD and progressive liver disease that eventually becomes irreversible.

But let's look a little bit deeper for a moment: Obesity is an inflammatory disease, as are heart disease and type 2 diabetes, the other components of metabolic syndrome.

And... you're probably way ahead of me now: Chronic inflammation dramatically elevates the production of free radical oxygen molecules, also forerunners of most of diseases of aging.

It's all starting to fall neatly into place now, don't you think?

Science Is On Your Side

The scientific evidence in favor of OPCs includes controlling inflammation, reversing free radical oxygen molecules, thereby helping prevent and reverse many types of disease, including all types of liver disease.

French grape seed extract supplements give you one of the most formidable tools science has against the negative health effects of obesity, a disease that is extremely difficult to treat and reverse.

In an impressive Saudi Arabian study, patients with fatty liver diseases, were given 100 mg of standardized grape seed extract for three months. Their liver function and liver enzymes greatly improved, including severely limiting the number of fat cells that were able to infiltrate the liver. Positive effects were even seen in patients given a small dose of only 50 mg daily.

Important animal studies from France and Spain confirm that overweight hamsters reduced their waistlines dramatically with grape seed extract, even when they were fed a high fat diet. In addition, the grape seed extract reduced blood sugars, increased the ability to use insulin produced by the pancreas and lowered blood fats—all important stepping stones to address metabolic syndrome and to eliminate and prevent heart disease and type 2 diabetes.

Exciting research published in the *Journal of Ethnopharmacology* shows that grape seed OPCs have another superpower rare in the plant world: they can cross the blood-brain barrier and maintain its ability to help regulate the hormones involved in hunger and satiety.

A Spanish animal study confirmed that grape seed extract protects against NAFLD and controls high cholesterol.

An impressive animal study from the University of Nevada at Reno showed grape seed extract is highly effective at reversing the effects of high triglycerides (fats in the bloodstream) that greatly increase the risk of heart disease. When researchers gave laboratory animals a super high fructose diet for eight weeks, all their triglyceride numbers shot up a frightening 171%! But animals given the same diet plus grape seed extract actually *reduced* their triglycerides by 41%.

Before we get too far with this line of thinking, we do want to note that grape seed extract is not a magic bullet. Taking French grape seed extract does not mean you neutralize all the negative effects of eating a highly processed diet by taking this powerful supplement.

The underlying causes of obesity and the ways to fight it could be the subject of several books but let me say that a healthy diet and an active lifestyle *plus* the powerhouse botanicals FGSE, andrographis, and milk thistle are highly effective botanicals that could quite literally save your life.

There's More . . .

FGSE has a well-earned place as one of science's most potent tools against chronic disease.

Only a handful of botanicals known today that can achieve these remarkable healing feats:

- Reduce inflammation, an underlying factor in many chronic diseases
- Lower blood pressure
- Strengthen and relax blood
- Lower cholesterol and triglycerides
- Control blood sugars
- Help reduce weight
- Protect brain cells
- Protect memory by helping create neural pathways as alternative pathways to transmit information
- Prevent and treat cancer (see more below)

Cancer is at the bottom of this list, but FGSE is an essential tool in cancer prevention and treatment as well. The OPCs in French grape seed extract have unique abilities to target cancer from several ways:

- Prevent carcinogenesis: Stop cells from becoming cancerous at all
- Inhibit tumorigenesis: Stop cancer cells from clumping together and forming cancerous tumors
- Promote apoptosis: Tell rapidly (and uncontrollably) reproducing cancer cells to return to their normal life cycles
- Inhibit angiogenesis: Stop tumors from building a blood supply to nourish and sustain themselves
- Reduce chemoresistance: Make conventional chemotherapy drugs more effective
- Inhibit metastasis: Stop cancer from spreading.

What's not to love about this multi-tasking botanical?

The Right Stuff

There are some cautions about grape seed extract, which is why we always recommend *French* grape seed extract. Many other (and often cheap) grape seed extract products can have high levels of tannins that are poorly absorbed and have few documented benefits. FGSE is the source of easily absorbable OPCs with the multitude of health benefits documented in this chapter and the reference section at the end of this book.

What You Need To Know:

French grape seed extract (FGSE) contains a wealth of oligomeric proanthocyanidins (OPCs), liver-protecting nutrients that science confirms:

- Control inflammation
- Reduce the production of disease-causing free radical oxygen molecules
- Promote weight loss
- Regulate production of brain chemicals that tell you "I'm full"
- Reduce inflammatory liver enzymes that lead to NAFLD, NASH, cirrhosis and liver cancer

Plus, OPCs have many other powerful health benefits:

- Prevent and treat cancer by attacking it in several ways
- Lower blood pressure
- Strengthen and relax blood vessel walls
- Lower cholesterol and triglycerides
- Control blood sugars
- Protect brain cells
- Protect memory by helping create neural pathways as alternative pathways to transmit information

CHAPTER 7
Milk Thistle

It would be impossible to talk about liver health without including milk thistle, often considered a weed. It's a weed with a host of medicinal benefits! Its pretty purple flowers and prickly leaves have been used to promote liver health for millennia.

Milk thistle (botanical name *Silybum marianum)* is related to the daisy and ragweed families. Although it is native to the Mediterranean countries, milk thistle is now found in many parts of the world, especially in warm, dry regions of North and South America. If you live in the United States, you are likely to find milk thistle sprouting in your garden.

Milk thistle is used to treat a wide range of liver diseases, including NAFLD, NASH, cirrhosis, and liver cancer. It offers what scientists call a "multi-targeted approach," which simply means it works in a wide variety of ways to protect and heal the liver.

Several studies show that silymarin, a group of flavonoid nutrients found in milk thistle seeds, has impressive anti-inflammatory and antioxidant powers and its ability to help the liver repel toxins that damage and destroy liver function.

Liver Protection

More than anything else, silymarin, is known as hepatoprotective or has the unique ability to protect liver cells from damage caused by a wide range of toxins. It shields liver cells from the barrage of free radicals, fats, sugars, and toxins that contribute to NAFLD and other liver ailments.

In previous chapters, we've taken a deep dive into the ways inflammation causes heart disease, type 2 diabetes and obesity, all of which are sometimes bundled into metabolic syndrome. We've also looked at the ways metabolic syndrome is closely connected to NAFLD.

Milk thistle joins the NAFLD fighting team as a powerful anti-inflammatory. It's also an important antioxidant that prevents cells from deteriorating and causing disease, including, of course, liver disease.

Overcoming Metabolic Syndrome

Silymarin has an active ingredient, silybin, that is credited with many of milk thistle's healing powers, beyond the impressive anti-inflammatory and antioxidant benefits. Italian research confirms that silybin blocks the accumulation of fat in the liver and can help reverse insulin resistance, an underlying cause of type 2 diabetes, a major risk factor for NAFLD.

If all that sounds complicated, it is. It's just important to know that silymarin and its jump starter, silybin, have a way to circle around liver disease, especially NAFLD, and fight it from several angles.

Here's another vicious circle: Liver disease can be the result of mitochondrial malfunction, which means that the cells just don't produce enough energy to do their jobs. Or mitochondrial malfunction may be caused by liver disease. It's a question of the chicken or the egg, but the effectiveness of milk thistle in preventing and even reversing NAFLD is clear. Plus, milk thistle is a powerful antioxidant that protects the mitochondria.

Slows Cirrhosis Progression

Perhaps the most impressive study we've found shows that milk thistle slows the progression of the deadly liver disease, cirrhosis. We know that cirrhosis is untreatable, but milk thistle has been proven to increase the lifespans of people with this end-stage liver disease. A pivotal Austrian study, published in 1989, showed that simple silymarin supplements increased the lifespans of people with cirrhosis. Without silymarin, only 39% survived for four years, but 58% who took silymarin survived for four years.

Fast Acting

Milk thistle works quickly. One study says it begins to reverse markers of NAFLD within two weeks. Turkish researchers found that milk thistle reversed all of the major markers for NAFLD: body and liver weights, lipid profiles, AST, ALT, and glucose levels.

In a groundbreaking study, researchers from the Czech Republic found that silymarin protected against the liver-destroying effects of acetaminophen (Tylenol™), one of the primary causes of poisoning worldwide.

Here's an interesting illustration of the power of milk thistle: It can neutralize the deadly attack on the liver if you accidentally eat a toxic mushroom like the deadly *Amanita phalloides* or the death cap mushroom. Aptly named, death caps can cause an agonizing death from liver failure.

Silymarin, if administered within minutes of ingesting a death cap mushroom, can completely neutralize the poison. If taken within 24 hours, it can minimize the liver toxicity, neurological impairment and even deaths (if given intravenously). This intravenous antidote has been licensed in Europe for many years and the Centers for Disease Control and Prevention confirmed in 2017 that it was investigating it as well.

NOTE: Never, ever eat wild mushrooms unless you are ***absolutely*** *sure of their identity*!

Excellent news: New formulations of silymarin and silybin have overcome absorbability problems and make its disease-fighting compounds easily available to the body with no serious side effects.

There's More . . .

Milk thistle has been lauded for more than 500 beneficial effects on the human body, including:

Antioxidant and anti-inflammatory:
It bears repeating: Milk thistle combats the free radical oxygen molecules that are the underlying cause of most diseases of aging, including heart disease, diabetes, cancer, and, yes, liver disease. It can even reduce the inflammation of chronic acne. This means milk thistle protects against these diseases and can help reverse them.

Antiviral:
Milk thistle is also used to help reduce the viral load in people with viral forms of hepatitis.

Improving blood sugars:
Chinese research confirms that silybin is at least as effective as the antidiabetic pharmaceutical, rosiglitazone, in controlling blood sugars. Plus, milk thistle is a much safer option, as some countries have pulled rosiglitazone from the market due to safety concerns.

Helping control weight:
Silybin has also been shown to target and reduce central obesity (abdominal fat) by helping break down fats and improving the body's ability to use glucose appropriately.

Cancer prevention:
Silymarin works several ways to protect against liver cancer as well as cancer of the breast, prostate, colon and lungs. It triggers apoptosis (programmed cell death preventing tumor growth), blocks invasion of healthy cells by cancerous cells, deprives cancerous tumors of the glucose they crave for energy, and triggers a wide range of cancer-suppressing genes.

Cancer treatment:
Some animal studies suggest it may minimize the side effects of chemotherapy and even make chemo work more effectively against certain types of cancer.

Breast milk production:
It can help make more prolactin, the milk-producing hormone in lactating women. One study suggests it can even dramatically increase the amount of milk that is produced. Note: while milk thistle is generally considered safe, pregnant or breast-feeding women should always consult their healthcare practitioner before starting any supplementation.

Memory and brain function:

It is known to protect against oxidative damage to the brain, prevent mental decline in aging and even reduce the number of amyloid plaques in animals with Alzheimer's disease.

Bone strength:

There are no human studies, but early research suggests that silymarin may stimulate the absorption of minerals needed to build strong bones and protect against bone loss, particularly in postmenopausal women.

What You Need to Know:

Milk thistle, its group of flavonoid ingredients, collectively named silymarin, containing the most active ingredient, silybin, have enormous protective and healing effects on the liver.

- Best known for protecting the liver against toxins that lead to NAFLD and NASH.
- Can help control weight, a primary factor in NAFLD.
- Can regulate blood sugar and reduce insulin resistance. Factors involved in type 2 diabetes and subsequent risk of NAFLD.
- Can stabilize cirrhosis of the liver, preventing progression to liver cancer and even death.
- Numerous other benefits, including protecting against several types of cancer, improving bone strength, and preserving memory and brain function.

CHAPTER 8
The Right Combo

From Terry Lemerond:

The last three chapters have given you a roadmap to botanicals that can help treat and even reverse some forms of liver disease.

In good conscience, I need to remind you that there is no magic wand or magic pill to treat or prevent liver disease. NAFLD and NASH are potentially reversible, but lifestyle changes must be the foundation of any plan to preserve or regain your liver health. In the simplest possible terms, this means prioritizing weight control, good nutrition and exercise.

You know yourself best. No one can tell you what will work best for you. The weight control plan that worked for your cousin or next-door neighbor may not be the solution for you. In Chapter 4, you got some tools for weight loss. we recommend you re-read that chapter and find what will work best for you.

Our personal recommendation is that you don't consider a weight loss program as a "diet." In fact, the word diet means the kinds of food that we habitually eat. Forming new habits can take time. That means aiming for slow and steady changes and weight loss.

A good starting point would be a restriction on sugar and simple carbohydrates (white bread, rice, pasta, etc.), while increasing fiber-rich and nutrient-dense foods like whole grains, fruits, healthy fats and non-starchy vegetables. The goal is to feel empowered in your choices and your health. That's the key to permanent weight control: You want to feel satisfied, fueled, and nourished.

All of that said, here's a further roadmap into the botanicals we discussed: andrographis, French grape seed extract and milk thistle to help you on the road to liver health.

What To Look For...

There are hundreds, perhaps thousands, of products on the market, while some of which may be helpful, some may not contain what they promise or contains cheap, ineffective ingredients. Some may make false promises, and some may even be harmful. It's essential to find the highest quality and most effective ingredients.

We know. That search can be overwhelming. We're here to help you make the right choices based on our combined decades of experience in the natural health industry, in addition to clinical education and experience.

Andrographis (*Andrographis paniculata*):
This is a powerful anti-inflammatory that can stop fibrosis that leads to dangerous cirrhosis. It can not only reverse, but also prevent, the progression of NAFLD. Look for a product that is standardized to 20% andrographolides to deliver 40 mg per capsule of this key compound for maximum benefits.

Recommended dosage: 200 mg twice daily of standardized andrographis

French grape seed extract (*Vitis vinifera*):
Remember that French grape seed is unlike any other grape seed extract available to protect liver cells from oxidative stress and damage. Look for a product that is tannin-free and contains 100% absorbable proanthocyanidins, standardized to contain 99% health promoting polyphenols.

Recommended dosage: 100 mg twice daily of French Grape Seed Extract standardized for polyphenol content.

Milk thistle (*Silybum marianum*):
This powerful anti-inflammatory protects your liver from a broad range of toxins and is one of nature's most effective tools against metabolic syndrome and liver disease. Look for a product that contains the fruit extract in a sunflower lecithin complex containing at least 29% of the most healing ingredient, silybin.

Recommended dosage: 100 mg twice daily.

The good news...

The authors of this book recommend taking these three herbal medicines together since they synergistically support one another for the treatment of the liver. Look for a formulation that includes all three online or at your health food store.

Supplements to take daily if you have NAFLD, NASH or cirrhosis:

- Andrographis: 200 mg, twice daily
- French grape seed extract: 100 mg, twice daily
- Milk thistle: 100 mg, twice daily

Please discuss these scientifically validated options with your healthcare practitioner(s), especially if you have already been diagnosed with liver disease. Feel free to copy this chapter and the next chapter in case your healthcare practitioner would like additional information on the healing power of these ingredients.

CHAPTER 9
Doc to Doc

Dear Readers: We all know our doctors and other healthcare professionals are very busy. As excited as you may be about this book and all it offers, it's unlikely you can persuade a medical professional to read the entire book. That's why we have written this information-packed and very concise summary of the book's contents specifically for people with scientific backgrounds. Many authors diligently protect their copyrights, but in this case, we encourage you to photocopy, scan or photograph the pages in this chapter and distribute them freely to healthcare professionals. You might want to include the reference section, so your practitioner can confirm the research mentioned here.

Dear HealthCare Professional,

Your patient has given you a copy of this chapter with my blessings and permission. My publisher and I have given it to the public domain so that the vital information it contains can be distributed freely. One of the goals is that medical professionals will become familiar with the value of these botanicals, scientifically validated to prevent and treat non-alcoholic fatty liver disease (NAFLD), NASH (non-alcoholic steatohepatitis), and even cirrhosis.

I understand that doctors are frequently skeptical about natural formulations and, if they haven't conducted their own investigations on a subject, they are inclined to steer their patients away from them, even though these formulations might be lifesaving. I urge you to spend a few minutes reviewing these few pages. Confirm them for yourself and consider adding them to your treatment options.

First let me introduce you to the three botanicals featured in the book:

Andrographis *(Andrographis paniculata)*:

An adaptogenic bitter, andrographis is widely used for colds, flu, and liver protection in Ayurvedic and Traditional Chinese Medicine (TCM). It is central to the herbal traditions of several Asian countries.

As is often the case, the effectiveness of a medicine that has been used and revered for millennia is now affirmed by modern science. By the end of 2022, the National Library of Medicine's database returned 1,242 published studies on the wide spectrum of health effects of andrographis dating as far back as 1951.

It's anti-inflammatory and antioxidant properties make andrographis an effective preventive and treatment for liver disease.

Many of the substantial healing powers of andrographis come from andrographolides, a rare group of diterpenoid lactones that have strong and scientifically proven anti-inflammatory, antioxidant, and antimicrobial effects. Andrographis is also a rich source of other nutrients, including well-researched antioxidant flavonoids and polyphenols.

In fact, andrographolide is so well regarded that pharmaceutical companies are even experimenting with synthetic versions.

Here's a summary of the most important published findings:

- Controls fibrosis and inflammation
- Reduces pro-inflammatory conditions, decreases liver enzyme values and liver fibrosis percentage
- Reverses AST and ALT markers (studied in obese lab animals)
- Reverses insulin resistance

A 2017 Indian study concluded, "Our results showed that (andrographolides) could be a promising lead to treat NAFLD with comparatively low toxicity and improved efficacy."

French grape seed extract *(Vitis vinifera)*:

The active compounds, oligomeric proanthocyanidins, in French grape seed extract (FGSE) are among the most potent antioxidants known to science. The substantial anti-inflammatory properties make it part of an ideal protocol for metabolic disorders like obesity, dyslipidemia, and NAFLD.

Here's a summary of the most important published findings:

- Clinical trials confirm improvements in liver enzymes of obese individuals given 100 mg of standardized grape seed extract daily
- Limits fat cell infiltration of the liver
- Reduces abdominal fat in animal studies, even when animals were fed a high fat diet
- Reduces blood glucose
- Improves insulin uptake
- Reduces triglycerides and cholesterol
- Positively influences the activity of leptin and ghrelin
- Crosses the blood-brain barrier and improves neural pathways

Milk thistle (*Silybum marianum)*:

Milk thistle is one of the most well-known and well-researched botanicals for liver health. Milk thistle is used to treat a wide range of liver diseases, including NAFLD, NASH, cirrhosis and liver cancer. It offers a multi-targeted approach to liver dysfunction.

Several studies show that silymarin, a group of flavonoid nutrients found in milk thistle seeds, has impressive anti-inflammatory and antioxidant powers. These benefits include an ability to help the liver repel toxins that damage and destroy liver function.

Here's a summary of the most important published findings:

- Hepatoprotective
- Blocks fat accumulation in the liver
- Reverses insulin resistance
- Silybin, an ingredient of silymarin, protects mitochondria
- Slows cirrhosis progression, extends life expectancy for patients with cirrhosis
- Reverses all major markers for NAFLD: body and liver weights, lipid profiles, AST and ALT, and glucose levels within two weeks
- Protects against acetaminophen toxicity
- New formulations have solved bioavailability issues

It makes sense to me that combining all of these botanicals will not only have a profound effect on your patients' liver health, they can also help stabilize and even reverse disease.

I'm sure you are well aware that there are questionable products on the market. Please consider the following recommendations from my experience.

Supplements for NAFLD or NASH:

- Andrographis: 200 mg
- French grape seed extract: 100 mg
- Milk thistle: 100 mg

Thanks for your attention and thanks in advance from your patients!

Lexi Loch, ND
Naturopathic physician
www.doclexiloch.com

References

Chapter 2: Liver Diseases

Agrawal S, Khazaeni B. Acetaminophen toxicity. https://www.ncbi.nlm.nih.gov/books/NBK441917/

Garcia-Chapman D, Jaquez-Quintana JO, Gonzalez-Gonzales JA et al. Liver cirrhosis and diabetes: Risk factors, pathophysiology, clinical implications and management. *World J Gastroenterol.* 2009 Jan 21; 15(3): 280–288.

Mirhafez SR, Dehabeh M, Hariri M et al. Curcumin and piperine combination for the treatment of patients with non-alcoholic fatty liver disease: A double-blind randomized placebo-controlled trial. *Adv Exp Med Biol.* 2021;1328:11-19.

Chapter 3: Non-Alcoholic Fatty Liver Disease

Yu EL, Schwimmer JB. Epidemiology of pediatric nonalcoholic fatty liver disease. *Clinical Liver Disease (Hoboken).* 2021;17(3):196–199.

Chalasani N, Younossi Z, Lavine JE, et al. The diagnosis and management of non-alcoholic fatty liver disease: practice guidance from the American Association for the Study of Liver Diseases. *Hepatology.* 2018;67(1):328–357.

Jung YK, Yim HJ. Reversal of liver cirrhosis: current evidence and expectations. *Korean J Intern Med.* 2017 Mar; 32(2): 213–228.

VanWagner LB, Armstrong MJ. Lean NAFLD: A not so benign condition? *Hepatol Commun.* 2018 Jan; 2(1): 5–8.

Chapter 4: How You Can Achieve A Healthy Liver

Puliese N, Torres MC et al. Is there an 'ideal' diet for patients with NAFLD? *Eur J Clin Invest.* 2022 Mar;52(3):e13659.

Sofi F, Casini A. Mediterranean diet and non-alcoholic fatty liver disease: new therapeutic option around the corner? *World J Gastroenterol.* 2014 Jun 21;20(23):7339-46.

Yin C, Li Z et al. Effect of intermittent fasting on non-alcoholic fatty liver disease: systematic review and meta-analysis. Front Nutr. 2021; 8: 709683.

Haghughatdoost F, Salehi-Abargouei A et al. The effects of low carbohydrate diets on liver function tests in nonalcoholic fatty liver disease: A systematic review and meta-analysis of clinical trials. J Res Med Sci. 2016; 21: 53.

Zelber-Sagi S, Buch A et al. Effect of resistance training on non-alcoholic fatty-liver disease a randomized-clinical trial. World J Gastroenterol. 2014 Apr 21; 20(15): 4382–4392.

Part 2: Botanicals to Promote Liver Health

Chapter 5: Andrographis

Dai Y, Chen SR et al. Overview of pharmacological activities of *Andrographis paniculata* and its major compound andrographolide. *Crit Rev Food Sci Nutr.* 2019;59(sup1):S17-S29.

Cabrera D, Wree A et al. Andrographolide ameliorates inflammation and fibrogenesis and attenuates inflammasome activation in experimental non-alcoholic steatohepatitis. Sci Rep. 2017; 7: 3491.

Li L, Li S,et al. Investigating pharmacological mechanisms of andrographolide on non-alcoholic steatohepatitis (NASH): A bioinformatics approach of network pharmacology. *Chin Herb Med.* 2021 Jul; 13(3): 342–350.

Chturvedi G.N., Tomar G.S., et al. 1983. Clinical studies on Kamesh (*Andrographis paniculata nees*) in infective hepatitis. *Anc Sci Life*. 2, 208–215.

Toppo E., Darvin, S. 2016. Effect of two andrographolide derivatives on cellular and rodent models of non-alcoholic fatty liver disease. *Molecules*. 21:8.

Bardi DA, Halabi MF, et al. *Andrographis paniculata* leaf extract prevents thioacetamide-induced liver cirrhosis in rats. *PLoS One.* 2014; 9(10): e109424.

Nagalekshmi R, Meno A et al. Hepatoprotective activity of *Andrographis paniculata* and *Swertia chirayita*. *Food Chem Toxicol.* 2011 Dec;49(12):3367-73.

Chapter 6: French Grape Seed Extract

Ardid-Ruiz A, Harazin A, Bama L, et al. The effects of *Vitis vinifera* L. phenolic compounds on a blood-brain barrier culture model: Expression of leptin receptors and protection against cytokine-induced damage.

Aguilar M, Bhuket T, et al. Prevalence of the metabolic syndrome in the United States, 2003-2012. Journal of the American Medical Association, *2015;* May 19;313(19):1973-4.

Sung KC, Rhee EJ, et al. Increased cardiovascular mortality in subjects with metabolic syndrome is largely attributable to diabetes and hypertension in 159,971 Korean adults. *Journal of Clinical Endocrinology and Metabolism,* 2015 Jul;100(7):2606-12.

Ogden CL, Carroll MD, et al. Prevalence of overweight and obesity in the United States, 1999-2004. *Journal of the American Medical Association,* 2006;295(13):1549-1555.

Sapwarobol S, et al. Postprandial blood glucose response to grape seed extract in healthy participants: A pilot study. *Pharmacogn Mag.* 2012;8(31):192-6.

Baskaran Y, Bhunvaneswari S, et al. Grape seed proanythocyanidins and metformin act by different mechanisms to promote insulin signaling in rats fed high calorie diet. *Journal of Cell Communication and Signaling.* 2013 Sep 12.

Caimari A, del Bas JM, et al. Low doses of grape seed procyanidins reduce adiposity and improve the plasma lipid profile in hamsters. *International Journal of Obesity* (London),2013 Apr;37(4):576-83.

Chapter 7: Milk Thistle

Gillessen A, Schmidt H. Silymarin as supportive treatment in liver diseases: a narrative review. *Adv Ther.* 2020; 37(4): 1279–1301.

Federico A, Dallio M, et al. Silymarin/silybin and chronic liver disease: a marriage of many years. *Molecules.* 2017 Jan 24;22(2):191.

Sornsuvit A, Hongwiset D, et al. The bioavailability and pharmacokinetics of silymarin smedds formulation study in healthy thai volunteers. *Evid Based Complement Alternat Med*. 2018; 2018: 1507834.

Yao J, Zhi M, et al. Effect of silybin on high-fat-induced fatty liver in rats. *Braz J Med Biol Res.* 2011 Jul;44(7):652-9.

Yaio J, Zhi M, et al. Effect and the probable mechanisms of silibinin in regulating insulin resistance in the liver of rats with non-alcoholic fatty liver. *Braz J Med Biol Res.* 2013 Mar;46(3):270-7.

Ferenci P, Dragosics B, et al. Randomized controlled trial of silymarin treatment in patients with cirrhosis of the liver. *J Hepatol.* 1989 Jul;9(1):105-13.

About the Authors

Terry Lemerond

Terry Lemerond is a natural health expert with over 50 years of experience helping people live healthier, happier lives. A much sought-after speaker and accomplished author, Terry shares his wealth of experience and knowledge in health and nutrition through his educational programs, including the Terry Talks Nutrition website TerryTalksNutrition.com—newsletters, pod- casts, webinars, and personal speaking engagements. Terry has also hosted Terry Talks Nutrition radio for the past 30 years. His books include:

Fight Disease With A Powerful Natural Seed–The Wonders of French Grape Seed Extract

Andrographis–The Natural Answer to Disease

Type 2 Diabetes? Break Free Naturally, with Hintonia

Wake UP! Melatonin is For More Than Just Sleep

Relieve Pain without Side Effects

Trauma Comfrey, Nature's Healing Herb

Drug-Free Relief of Anxiety & Stress

Propolis, The Natural Way to Prevent and Heal Infection: Fights Infection Including: Bacterial, Viral, Fungal, Parasitic, and More

The Wise Ginseng Choice for Restored Health- HRG80™ Red Ginseng: The powerful answer to: Lack of Energy, Fatigue, Exhaustion, Cancer, Diabetes, Alzheimer's and more, Sexual Performance

Polyphenol Power! Polyphenols in fruit and vegetables to prevent and cure: Heart Disease, Cancer, Type 2 Diabetes, Alzheimer's and more!

Outsmart Cancer With Powerful Natural Medicines

THE MEDITERRANEAN ANTI-AGING SECRET TO VIBRANT HEALTH
Greek Mountain Tea is the Ancient Secret to:•Improved Mental Clarity
•Reduced Anxiety •Strong Immunity •Bone Density •Preventing Alzheimer's Disease

50+ Natural Health Secrets Proven to Change Your Life

Discovering Your Best Health

How To Improve Your Health at Any Age

Seven Keys to Vibrant Health

Seven Keys to Unlimited Personal Achievement

Terry continues to author and co-author books to educate everyone on the steps they can take to live a healthier, vibrant life.

His continual dedication, energy, and zeal are part of his ongoing mission—to help us all improve our health.

Dr. Lexi Loch

Dr. Lexi Loch received her doctorate in naturopathic medicine from the National University of Natural Medicine, where she graduated with highest honors.

In addition to her practice, she is a medical writer and editor, researcher, educator, and patient advocate. Her articles have been published in various natural health periodicals and reference books.

More about TTN Publishing, LLC

Everyone has the same desire:
a vibrant, healthy life!

Everyone has the same desire: a vibrant, healthy life!

TTN Publishing exists to provide educational information anyone can use to understand how herbs and botanical medicines play a vital role in optimal health. From a stomachache to a life-threatening disease, even cancer, the plant kingdom has safe, effective phytonutrients and answers for healthy living.

Author and health pioneer Terry Lemerond brings his vast knowledge of plant medicines combined with cutting edge research from today's top scientists and doctors directly to consumers.

Each TTN Publishing, LLC book is crafted to provide the necessary basic information and recommendations for how botanicals can be used in practical ways to fight disease and improve the path to healthy living.

Education, information, scientific validation, and common sense are a part of every TTN Publishing endeavor. There are many books to come, so stay connected! With 80 percent of the world's population depending on plant medicines, you can join in the knowledge and wisdom available to meet your health goals.

Welcome to TTN Publishing!

We'd love to hear from you!

info@ttnpublishing.com

www.TTNPublishing.com

Would you like to be one of the first to know the latest updates on Terry's books?

- Learn more about his background and new
- books
- See photos, videos, and the latest news
- Listen to Terry's radio show and podcasts, including archived programs on a multitude of subjects
- Sign up for a free weekly email newsletter and educational webinar notices

It's all available at www.TerryTalksNutrition.com

Don't forget to connect at:
www.facebook.com/TerryTalksNutrition

Visit and follow Terry's author page on Amazon:
www.amazon.com/author/terrylemerond

Share this exciting news!

If you appreciated this book, please let others know.

- Pick up another copy and share with a friend
- Talk about it on social media
- Write a review on your blog or website
- Recommend this book to friends and family

Thank you for being a true health seeker!

Also by Terry Lemerond and available on Amazon

(Free in Kindle Unlimited and available in eBook and paperback)

Fight Disease with a Powerful, Natural Seed – The Wonders of French Grape Seed Extract
Prevent and Reverse: Cancer, Heart Disease, Diabetes, Alzheimer's & More
by Terry Lemerond and Ajay Goel M.S. Ph.D.
https://www.amazon.com/Fight-Disease-Powerful-Natural-Seed-ebook/dp/B08MB12PF9

Andrographis: The Natural Answer to Disease
Protection Against: Colds, flu, & upper respiratory infections, joint pain and arthritis, diabetes, heart disease, liver disease, cancer, and much more!
by Terry Lemerond and Alexander Panossian, Ph.D.
https://www.amazon.com/ANDROGRAPHIS-NATURAL-DISEASE-Terry-Lemerond-ebook/dp/B08T9XS846

Type 2 Diabetes? Break Free Naturally with Hintonia
by Terry Lemerond and Jacob Teitelbaum, M.D.
https://www.amazon.com/Type-Diabetes-Break-Naturally-Hintonia-ebook/dp/B08ZT3TVP4

Relieve Pain Without Side Effects: You Can Be Pain-free, Naturally!
by Terry Lemerond and Jan McBarron M.D.
https://www.amazon.com/Relieve-Pain-Without-Side-Effects-ebook/dp/B091QCJW51

Wake UP! Melatonin is For More Than Just Sleep
by Terry Lemerond and a forward by Jacob Teitelbaum, M.D
https://www.amazon.com/Wake-Melatonin-More-Than-Sleep-ebook/dp/B092KZHR88

Trauma Comfrey, Nature's Healing Herb
by Terry Lemerond and Holly Lucille, ND, RN
https://www.amazon.com/Trauma-Comfrey-Natures-Healing-Herb-ebook/dp/B09JWRMCLJ

Drug-Free Relief of Anxiety & Stress
by Terry Lemerond and Dr. Lynn Wagner
https://www.amazon.com/Drug-Free-Relief-Anxiety-Stress-Stress-Induced-ebook/dp/B09JWVQV18

Propolis The Natural Way to Prevent and Heal Infection: Fights Infection Including: Bacterial, Viral, Fungal, Parasitic, and More
by Terry Lemerond
https://www.amazon.com/Propolis-Natural-Prevent-Heal-Infection/dp/1952507227

The Wise Ginseng Choice for Restored Health-HRG80™ Red Ginseng: The powerful answer to: Lack of Energy, Fatigue, Exhaustion, Cancer, Diabetes, Alzheimer's and more, Sexual Performance
by Terry Lemerond and Jacob Teitelbaum MD
https://www.amazon.com/Ginseng-Choice-Restored-HRG80TM-GINSENG-ebook/dp/B0B6QDQLGS

Polyphenol Power! Polyphenols in fruit and vegetables to prevent and cure: Heart Disease, Cancer, Type 2 Diabetes, Alzheimer's and more!
by Terry Lemerond
https://www.amazon.com/POLYPHENOL-POWER-Polyphenols-vegetables-Alzheimers-ebook/dp/B0B6Q7GS9F

Outsmart Cancer With Powerful Natural Medicines
By Terry Lemerond, Ajay Goel, Ph.D., AGAF
https://www.amazon.com/Outsmart-Cancer-POWERFUL-NATURAL-MEDICINES-ebook/dp/B0C6X7NQ5Q

THE MEDITERRANEAN ANTI-AGING SECRET TO VIBRANT HEALTH
Greek Mountain Tea is the Ancient Secret to:
•Improved Mental Clarity •Reduced Anxiety
•Strong Immunity •Bone Density •Preventing Alzheimer's Disease
https://www.amazon.com/MEDITERRANEAN-ANTI-AGING-SECRET-VIBRANT-HEALTH-ebook/dp/B0C5KFXSF6

Additional paperback books:

Terry Talks Nutrition 50+ Natural Health Secrets Proven to Change Your Life
https://www.amazon.com/Nutrition-Natural-Secrets-resource-natural/dp/1732195900

Discovering Your Best Health
How To Improve Your Health at Any Age
https://www.amazon.com/Discovering-Your-Best-Health-IMPROVE/dp/1952507316

Made in the USA
Monee, IL
13 September 2026

62980099R00069